IBS DIET COOKBOOK FOR BEGINNERS

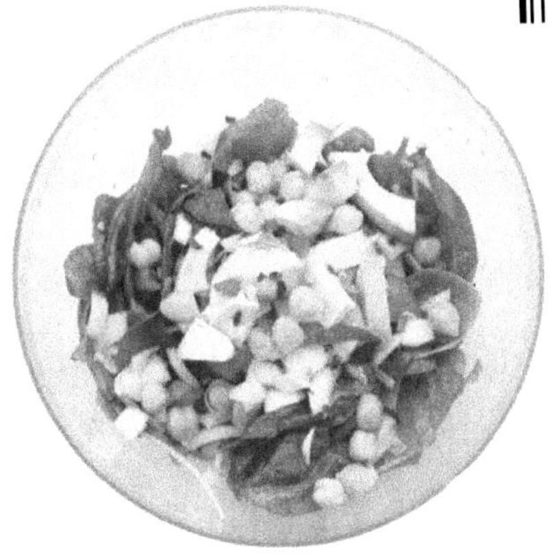

"Nourishing and Balanced Meals for IBS Relief"

Allie Nagel

Copyright © 2023 by Allie Nagel

DISCLAIMER

This cookbook is intended to provide general information and recipes. The recipes provided in this cookbook are not intended to replace or be a substitute for medical advice from a physician.

The reader should consult a healthcare professional for any specific medical advice, diagnosis or treatment.

Any specific dietary advice provided in this cookbook is not intended to replace or be a substitute for medical advice from a physician.

The author is not responsible or liable for any adverse effects experienced by readers of this cookbook as a result of following the recipes or dietary advice provided.

The author makes no representations or warranties of any kind (express or implied) as to the accuracy, completeness, reliability or suitability of the recipes provided in this cookbook.

The author disclaims any and all liability for any damages arising out of the use or misuse of the recipes provided in this cookbook.

The reader must also take care to ensure that the recipes provided in this cookbook are prepared and cooked safely. The recipes provided in this cookbook are for informational purposes only and should not be used as a substitute for professional medical advice, diagnosis or treatment.

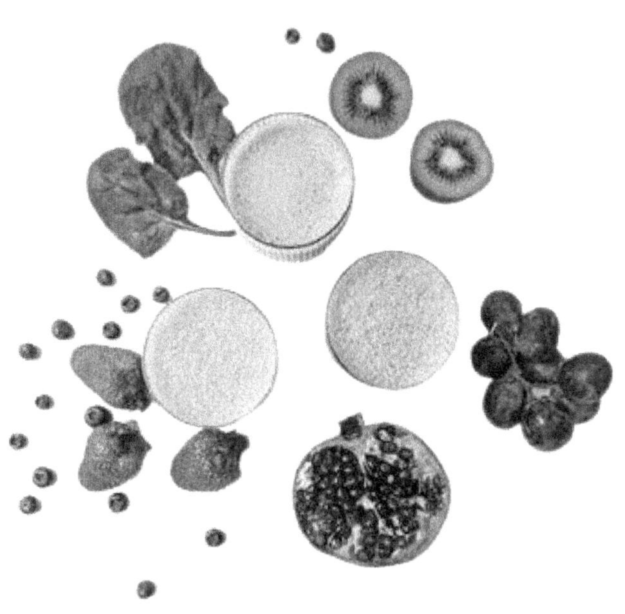

TABLE OF CONTENTS

INTRODUCTION

Maria's life was a constant battle. Every day, she faced an invisible enemy that tormented her from within.

Irritable Bowel Syndrome (IBS) had taken hold of her, wreaking havoc on her body and mind.

The excruciating pain, bloating, and unpredictable bowel movements had become her cruel companions, leaving her feeling isolated and hopeless.

Maria's IBS had turned her life into a nightmare. Social gatherings became a source of anxiety rather than joy.

The fear of an embarrassing incident or sudden flareup overshadowed every moment of happiness.

She had lost count of the countless nights spent curled up in agony, crying herself to sleep, wondering if her life would ever be normal again.

Feeling desperate, Maria decided it was time to take matters into her own hands.

She delved into research, seeking any glimmer of hope that could provide her with relief. That's when she stumbled upon a ray of light, the potential of dietary changes.

With newfound determination, Maria embarked on a journey of selfdiscovery through her kitchen.

She bid farewell to processed foods, greasy fast food, and excessive sugar. Instead, she embraced whole, unprocessed foods and carefully selected ingredients that were gentle on her delicate digestive system.

The results were astounding. Slowly but surely, Maria's body began to respond positively. The pain lessened and her once bloated belly started to flatten.

Gone were the days of running to the restroom in a panic; instead, she enjoyed a newfound sense of control over her body.

As Maria's physical health improved, so did her emotional wellbeing. The weight of IBS lifted from her shoulders, and she rediscovered the joys of socializing and connecting with loved ones.

If you too find yourself trapped in the clutches of IBS, take heart in Maria's story. There is hope and relief is within reach.

CHAPTER 1

UNDERSTANDING IBS AND ITS DIETARY IMPLICATIONS

What is Irritable Bowel Syndrome (IBS)?

Irritable Bowel Syndrome (IBS) is a common disorder that affects the large intestine (colon).

It is characterized by a group of symptoms that can vary in severity and duration, including abdominal pain, bloating, changes in bowel habits (such as diarrhea or constipation), and a sense of incomplete bowel movements.

The exact cause of IBS is not known, but it is believed to involve a combination of factors, including abnormal muscle contractions in the intestines, increased sensitivity to pain in the digestive system, and disturbances in the communication between the brain and the gut.

IBS is a chronic condition, meaning it is ongoing and often lasts for a long time. It can have a significant impact on a person's quality of life, causing discomfort, distress, and affecting daily activities.

The symptoms of IBS can be triggered or worsened by various factors, such as certain foods, stress, hormonal changes, and infections.

Diagnosing IBS involves a process of elimination, as there is no specific test to definitively diagnose the condition.

A healthcare provider will typically consider the patient's symptoms, medical history, and conduct tests to rule out other possible causes of the symptoms.

Treatment for IBS focuses on managing the symptoms and may involve a combination of lifestyle changes, dietary modifications, stress management techniques, and medications to alleviate specific symptoms.

Moreso, it's important for individuals with IBS to work closely with their healthcare provider to develop a personalized treatment plan.

Identifying Common Triggers and Symptoms

Triggers of Irritable Bowel Syndrome:

Food intolerances: Certain foods such as dairy products, gluten, caffeine, and artificial sweeteners may trigger IBS symptoms in some individuals.

Stress: Emotional stress and anxiety can exacerbate IBS symptoms or act as a trigger.

Hormonal changes: Fluctuations in hormone levels, particularly in women during their menstrual cycles, can contribute to IBS symptoms.

Medications: Certain medications, such as antibiotics, can disrupt the gut microbiota and trigger IBS symptoms.

Infection: A previous gastrointestinal infection, such as gastroenteritis, can increase the risk of developing IBS.

Changes in routine: Disruptions in regular meal times, sleep patterns, or travel can trigger IBS symptoms.

Alcohol and caffeine: Consumption of alcoholic or caffeinated beverages can stimulate the intestines and worsen IBS symptoms.

Large meals: Eating large, heavy meals can put additional strain on the digestive system and lead to IBS symptoms.

Gasproducing foods: Certain foods, such as beans, lentils, cabbage, and onions, can produce excess gas and trigger discomfort in individuals with IBS.

Lack of physical activity: Sedentary lifestyles and lack of exercise can contribute to IBS symptoms.

Symptoms of Irritable Bowel Syndrome:

Abdominal pain or cramping: Recurrent episodes of abdominal pain or cramping are common in individuals with IBS. The pain often improves after a bowel movement.

Changes in bowel habits: IBS can cause alterations in bowel movements, such as diarrhea, constipation, or a combination of both (alternating diarrhea and constipation).

Bloating and excessive gas: Many people with IBS experience bloating, which is the feeling of increased abdominal fullness or distension. This can be accompanied by increased gas production and flatulence.

Urgency to have a bowel movement: IBS can lead to a sudden and urgent need to have a bowel movement, often followed by relief after emptying the bowels.

Mucus in the stool: Some individuals with IBS may notice the presence of mucus in their stool, which is a gellike substance.

Fatigue and reduced energy levels: Chronic IBS symptoms can cause fatigue and a general feeling of low energy.

Nausea and vomiting: IBS may be associated with occasional episodes of nausea and vomiting, although these symptoms are less common.

Anxiety and depression: The chronic nature of IBS and its impact on daily life can contribute to anxiety and depression in some individuals.

Backache: Some people with IBS may experience lower back pain, which can be associated with the abdominal discomfort.

Sleep disturbances: Sleep problems, such as insomnia or restless sleep, can occur in individuals with IBS, often due to discomfort or frequent bowel movements during the night.

10 Benefits of IBS Relief Diet

1. Symptom relief: An IBS diet can help reduce the frequency and severity of IBS symptoms such as abdominal pain, bloating, gas, diarrhea, and constipation.

2. Improved digestion: By avoiding trigger foods that may aggravate the digestive system, an IBS diet can promote better digestion and alleviate digestive discomfort.

3. Enhanced bowel regularity: A wellbalanced IBS diet can help regulate bowel movements, reducing the occurrence of diarrhea or constipation associated with IBS.

4. Reduced inflammation: Some components of an IBS diet, such as fiberrich foods and omega3 fatty acids, can have antiinflammatory effects, which may help reduce inflammation in the gut.

5. Balanced gut microbiota: An IBS diet often includes prebioticrich foods that support the growth of beneficial gut bacteria, promoting a healthier gut microbiota and potentially reducing IBS symptoms.

6. Increased nutrient intake: By following an IBS diet, individuals can focus on consuming nutrientdense foods that provide essential vitamins, minerals, and antioxidants necessary for overall health.

7. Weight management: An IBS diet that emphasizes whole, unprocessed foods can support healthy weight management by providing a balanced intake of calories and nutrients.

8. Improved energy levels: By avoiding trigger foods and consuming a wellrounded diet, individuals may experience improved energy levels, reduced fatigue, and enhanced overall wellbeing.

9. Enhanced quality of life: When IBS symptoms are effectively managed through a suitable diet, individuals may experience a significant improvement in their quality of life, including reduced stress and anxiety related to digestive symptoms.

10. Personalized approach: An IBS diet often involves identifying individual trigger foods through an elimination and reintroduction process, allowing individuals to tailor their diet to their specific needs and gain a better understanding of their body's response to different foods.

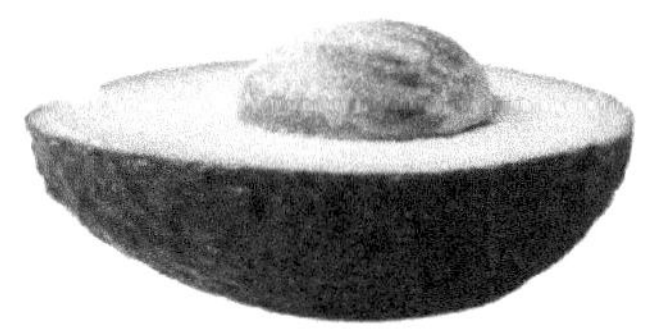

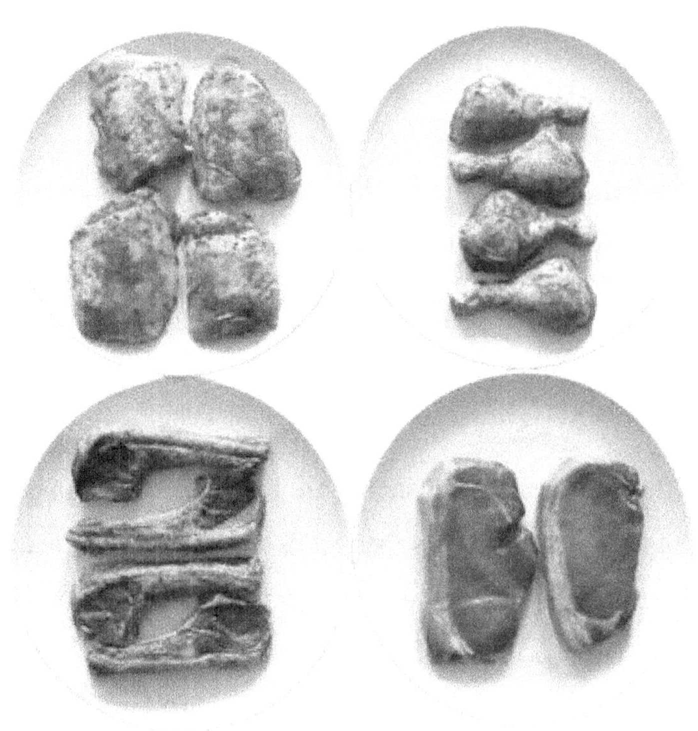

CHAPTER 2

Meal Plan

DAY 1

Breakfast: Oatmeal with almond milk and nuts

Lunch: Salmon and Avocado Salad

Dinner: Baked Salmon with Asparagus

DAY 2

Breakfast: Smoothie made with banana and walnuts

Lunch: Turkey Mason Jar Salad

Dinner: Broiled Chicken with Steamed Veggies

DAY 3

Breakfast: Poached eggs on toast with avocado

Lunch: Avocado and spinach Salad

Dinner: Slow Cooker Turkey Chili

DAY 4

Breakfast: Buckwheat pancakes

Lunch: Miso Soup with Cubed Tofu

Dinner: Zucchini Noodles with Tomato Sauce

DAY 5

Breakfast: Coconut porridge with chia seeds

Lunch: Egg Drop Soup

Dinner: Greek Egg & Vegetable Bake

DAY 6

Breakfast: Baked egg plant with almond butter

Lunch: Probiotic Veggie Wrap

Dinner: Spinach & Cauliflower Risotto

DAY 7

Breakfast: Carrot and ginger muffins

Lunch: Avocado Toast with Eggs

Dinner: Turkey & Vegetable Meatloaf

DAY 8

Breakfast: Tofu scramble with kale and avocado

Lunch: Sauteed Spinach and Mushrooms

Dinner: Broiled Cod with Herbed Brown Rice

DAY 9

Breakfast: Steel cut oats with mashed banana and coconut flakes

Lunch: Zucchini Frittata

Dinner: Oven Roasted Turkey & Vegetables

DAY 10

Breakfast: Scrambled eggs with zucchini and ginger foots herbs

Lunch: Egg omelet with whole wheat bread

Dinner: Roasted Vegetable & Tuna

DAY 11

Breakfast: Oatmeal with almond milk and nuts

Lunch: Salmon and Avocado Salad

Dinner: Baked Salmon with Asparagus

DAY 12

Breakfast: Smoothie made with banana and walnuts

Lunch: Turkey Mason Jar Salad

Dinner: Broiled Chicken with Steamed Veggies

DAY 13

Breakfast: Poached eggs on toast with avocado

Lunch: Avocado and spinach Salad

Dinner: Slow Cooker Turkey Chili

DAY 14

Breakfast: Buckwheat pancakes

Lunch: Miso Soup with Cubed Tofu

Dinner: Zucchini Noodles with Tomato Sauce

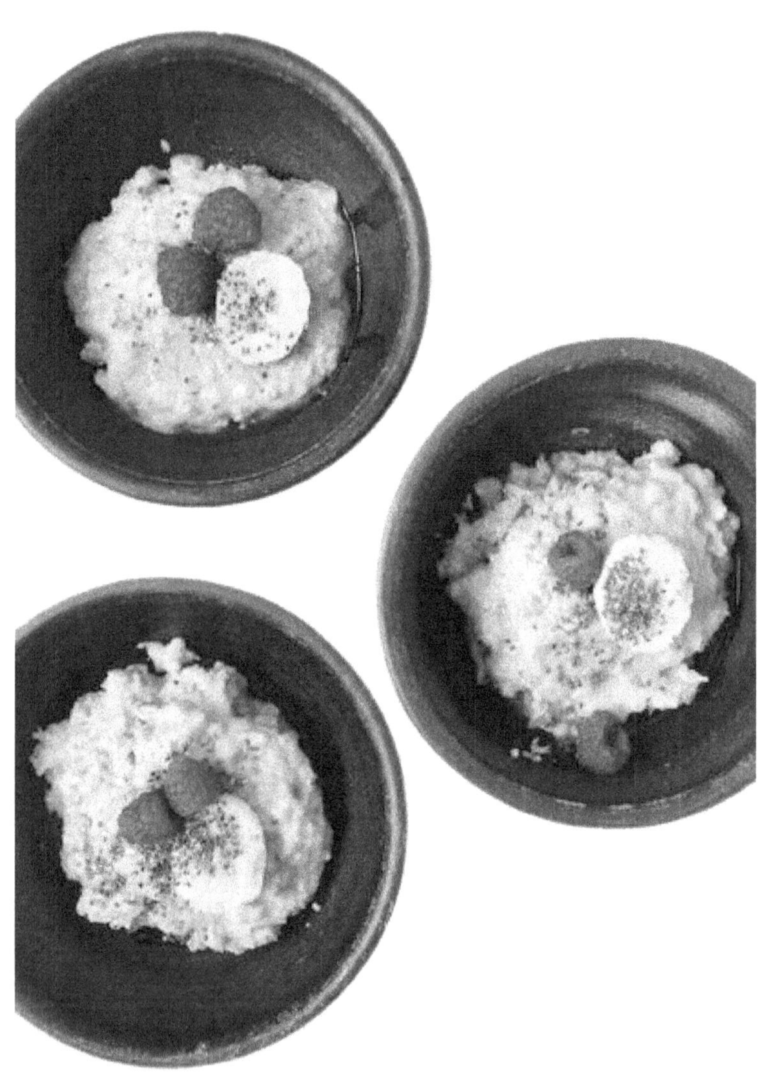

CHAPTER 3

30 IBSFriendly Recipes

BREAKFAST

Oatmeal with almond milk and nuts

Start your day off right with this nutritious and tasty oatmeal, packed with healthy fiber and antioxidants found in almonds that are particularly beneficial for those with Irritable bowel syndrome.

Ingredients:

1 cup oats

2 cups almond milk

1/4 cup chopped nuts (almonds, walnuts, pecans, or hazelnuts work best)

Optional: honey, dried fruits, cinnamon, nutmeg

Method of Preparation:

1. Bring the almond milk to a gentle boil in a mediumsized pot over medium heat.

2. Once boiling, add the oats to the pot and stir.

3. Reduce the heat to low and let the oats cook for 57 minutes, stirring occasionally until the oats reach your desired consistency.

4. Take the pot off the heat and stir in the chopped nuts and any desired additional flavorings.

5. Serve the oatmeal with a sprinkle of nuts and any additional desired toppings.

Preparation Time: 10 minutes

Serving Suggestion: Serve with fresh fruit such as banana, berries or apples.

Smoothie made with banana and walnuts

Enjoy a sweet smoothie made with banana and walnuts together to give you a boost of energy helping ward off IBS symptoms thanks to the magnesium found in walnuts.

Ingredients:

1 banana

1 cup almond milk

1/4 cup walnuts

Optional: dates, honey, cinnamon, nutmeg

Method of Preparation:

1. Place all the ingredients into a blender.

2. Blend until smooth.

Preparation Time: 5-10 minutes

Serving Suggestion: Serve with a sprinkle of cocoa powder or crushed nuts.

Poached eggs on toast with avocado

This delicious dinner option has plenty of health benefits that can help ease the symptoms of IBS with its high fiber and antioxidant content found in the avocado.

Ingredients:

2 eggs

2 slices of toast

1/4 tsp white wine vinegar or lemon juice

1/4 avocado, peeled and sliced

Optional: salt and pepper, chili flakes

Method of Preparation:

1. Fill a mediumsized saucepan halfway with water and bring to a gentle simmer.

2. Add the vinegar or lemon juice to the saucepan.

3. Carefully crack each egg into the saucepan, one at a time.

4. Allow the eggs to poach for 4 minutes, or until the whites are cooked and the yolks are still runny.

5. Meanwhile, toast the bread slices.

6. Once the eggs are cooked, remove them with a slotted spoon and place on top of the toast slices.

7. Top with avocado slices, and season with salt and pepper and chili flakes, if desired.

Preparation Time: 15 minutes

Serving Suggestion: Serve with a side salad.

Buckwheat pancakes

Make these deliciously fluffy pancakes that are packed with minerals like manganese, copper and phosphorus which can reduce inflammation and support bowel movement regularity.

Ingredients:

1 cup buckwheat flour

½ tsp baking powder

1 cup almond milk

1 egg

1 Tbsp honey

Optional: ½ tsp cinnamon, 1 Tbsp melted coconut oil

Method of Preparation:

1. In a mediumsized bowl, whisk together the buckwheat flour and baking powder.

2. Add the almond milk, egg and honey and whisk until combined.

3. If desired, add the coconut oil and cinnamon and whisk until everything is combined.

4. Heat a nonstick skillet over medium heat and grease lightly with butter or oil.

5. Ladle about ¼ cup of the batter onto the skillet and cook for 23 minutes until the edges start to bubble and the bottom is golden brown.

6. Flip and cook the other side for an additional 23 minutes.

7. Transfer the cooked pancakes to a plate and continue with the remaining batter.

Preparation Time: 15 minutes

Serving Suggestion: Serve with fresh fruit and a drizzle of honey or maple syrup.

Coconut porridge with chia seeds

Enjoy a filling breakfast with this coconut porridge for a rich and creamy texture with chia seeds for an additional punch of antioxidants to ease IBS symptoms.

Ingredients:

1 cup rolled oats

2 cups coconut milk

2 Tbsp chia seeds

Optional: honey, cinnamon, dried fruits

Method of Preparation:

1. In a mediumsized saucepan, bring the coconut milk to a gentle simmer over medium heat.

2. Slowly add the rolled oats and chia seeds and stir until combined.

3. Reduce the heat to low and let the porridge cook for 10 minutes, stirring occasionally, until the oats have reached your desired consistency.

4. Turn off the heat and stir in any desired additional flavorings.

Preparation Time: 15 minutes

Serving Suggestion: Serve with banana slices and a drizzle of honey or maple syrup.

Baked eggplant with almond butter

Enjoy this savory dish bursting with flavor and nutrition. Eggplant is packed with antioxidants, vitamins and minerals while the almond butter provides healthy fiber and healthy fats to help sooth IBS symptoms.

Ingredients:

1 large eggplant, diced

2 Tbsp almond butter

Optional: honey, lime juice, garlic powder, salt and pepper

Method of Preparation:

1. Preheat the oven to 375°F.

2. Place the diced eggplant on a greased baking sheet and spread with the almond butter.

3. Sprinkle with desired additional seasonings.

4. Bake for 2025 minutes until the eggplant is tender.

Preparation Time: 25 minutes

Serving Suggestion: Serve with a side salad or roasted vegetables.

Carrot and ginger muffins

These glutenfree muffins are packed with a powerful combination of vitamins and minerals from the carrots and ginger that can help manage the symptoms of IBS.

Ingredients:

3/4 cups allpurpose flour

3/4 cups whole wheat flour

1 teaspoon baking powder

1 teaspoon ground ginger

1/4 teaspoon ground nutmeg

1/2 teaspoon sea salt

3/4 cup coconut sugar

2/3 cup canola oil

2 eggs

2 1/2 cups grated carrot

Optional: 1/4 cup chopped walnuts

Method of Preparation:

1. Preheat the oven to 350°F. Grease a 12cup muffin pan.

2. In a mediumsized bowl, whisk together the flours, baking powder, ginger, nutmeg and salt.

3. In a separate bowl, whisk together the coconut sugar, canola oil, and eggs until combined.

4. Fold in the grated carrot.

5. Add the dry ingredients and mix until just combined.

6. Spoon the batter into the prepared muffin pan, filling each cup about 3/4 full.

7. Bake for 20-25 minutes or until a toothpick inserted into the center comes out clean.

8. Allow the muffins to cool before serving.

Preparation Time: 30 minutes

Serving Suggestion: Serve with a spread of almond butter and a cup of tea.

Tofu scramble with kale and avocado

This vegan breakfast won't leave you hungry with its high protein and fiber content from the tofu, kale and avocado. All these key nutrients can help ease IBS symptoms.

Ingredients:

1 block tofu, crumbled

1/2 cup kale, roughly chopped

1/4 avocado, peeled and diced

Air fryer cup mattymek

Optional: 1/2 tsp turmeric, chili flakes, garlic powder

Method of Preparation:

1. Heat a large nonstick skillet over medium heat and add the crumbled tofu.

2. Add the kale and desired seasonings and stir to combine.

3. Cook, stirring occasionally, until the tofu is golden brown and the kale has softened.

4. Add in the diced avocado and cook for an additional 12 minutes.

Preparation Time: 10 minutes

Serving Suggestion: Serve with a side of toast or roasted vegetables.

Steel cut oats with mashed banana and coconut flakes

High in soluble fiber, this breakfast can help you feel fuller for longer reducing the chances of an IBS flareup while the banana and coconut flakes offer a sweet flavor.

Ingredients:

1/2 cup steel cut oats

3/4 cup almond milk

1 banana, mashed

1/4 cup shredded coconut

Optional: 1/2 tsp cinnamon, 1 Tbsp honey

Method of Preparation:

1. Bring the almond milk to a boil in a mediumsized pot over medium heat.

2. Once boiling, reduce the heat to low and stir in the steel cut oats.

3. Cook the oats for 1520 minutes until the oats reach your desired consistency.

4. Take the pot off the heat and stir in the mashed banana, shredded coconut and any desired additional seasonings.

Preparation Time: 20 minutes

Serving Suggestion: Serve with a sprinkle of toasted nuts and a drizzle of honey or maple syrup.

Scrambled eggs with zucchini and ginger foots herbs

This tasty and nutritious breakfast will give your digestive system some breathing room with its high fiber content from the zucchini as well as the immunityboosting benefits of ginger and herbs which can help ease IBS symptoms.

Ingredients:

2 eggs

1/2 cup grated zucchini

1 Tbsp fresh ginger, minced

2 Tbsp fresh herbs (parsley, chives or dill work well)

Optional: salt and pepper, 1 Tbsp olive oil

Method of Preparation:

1. Heat a nonstick skillet over medium heat.

2. Add the eggs to the pan and scramble until the whites are just set.

3. Add the grated zucchini, ginger and herbs and stir to combine.

4. If desired, season with salt and pepper and drizzle with olive oil.

Preparation Time: 10 minutes

Serving Suggestion: Serve with a side of roasted potatoes or fresh toast.

LUNCH

Salmon and Avocado Salad

This salad is a nutritious combination of omega3rich salmon and fiberfilled avocado, making it a great meal choice for those with irritable bowel syndrome.

Ingredients:

 4 ounces grilled salmon (or tuna), cut into small cubes

2 small avocados, sliced

Juice of 1 lime

1/4 teaspoon salt

1/4 teaspoon freshly ground pepper

4 cups mixed greens of your choice

2 tablespoons olive oil

Preparation Time: 10 minutes

Method of Preparation:

1. Start by preparing the salmon (or tuna) by grilling it for a few minutes until cooked through. Allow to cool slightly before cutting into small cubes.

2. Slice the avocados and place them in a medium mixing bowl. Squeeze the lime juice on top and season with the salt and pepper. Gently toss to combine.

3. Add the mixed greens into the bowl and drizzle with the olive oil. Toss until evenly mixed.

4. Finally, add the cubed salmon and gently mix everything together.

Serving Suggestions: Enjoy this salad as a light lunch or dinner with a side of quinoa or brown rice.

Turkey Mason Jar Salad

This delicious and healthy mason jar salad combines lean turkey and a variety of highfiber fresh veggies for an easily transportable meal that is beneficial for those with IBS.

Ingredients:

2 tablespoons balsamic vinaigrette

4 ounces roast turkey breast, cubed

1/4 cup roasted red peppers, chopped

1/4 cup cherry tomatoes, halved

1/4 cup cucumber, diced

1/4 cup feta cheese

2 cups mixed greens of your choice

Preparation Time: 10 minutes

Method of Preparation:

1. Begin by adding 2 tablespoons of balsamic vinaigrette to a wide mouth mason jar.

2. Next, layer the salad ingredients in the jar in the following order: cubed turkey, roasted red peppers, cherry tomatoes, cucumber, feta cheese and lastly, the mixed greens.

3. Screw the lid on the jar and shake it up until the ingredients are well combined.

4. When ready to eat, pour the contents onto a plate and enjoy!

Serving Suggestions: Enjoy this salad as a light lunch or dinner with a side of quinoa or brown rice.

Avocado and Spinach Salad

This meal is bursting with vitaminrich ingredients, such as avocados, spinach, sunflower seeds, and garlic, all of which are key contributors to good digestive health.

Ingredients:

2 small avocados, diced

2 cups baby spinach

Juice of 1 lemon

1/4 teaspoon salt

1/4 teaspoon freshly ground pepper

2 tablespoons olive oil

Preparation Time: 10 minutes

Method of Preparation:

1. Begin by slicing the avocados into small cubes and transfer to a medium mixing bowl.

2. Add the baby spinach to the bowl.

3. Squeeze the lemon juice on top and season with the salt and pepper.

4. Drizzle the olive oil over the salad and toss until evenly mixed.

Serving Suggestions: Enjoy this salad as a light lunch or dinner with a side of quinoa or brown rice.

Miso Soup with Cubed Tofu

Enjoy this miso soup, made with highprotein cubed tofu and probioticrich miso, for a delicious and beneficial meal choice for those suffering from IBS.

Ingredients:

2 tablespoons white miso paste

3 cups vegetable broth

3/4 cup cubed firm tofu

1/2 cup sliced shiitake mushrooms

2 scallions, sliced

1 tablespoon sesame oil

Preparation Time: 10 minutes

Method of Preparation:

1. Begin by adding the white miso paste to a medium pot with the vegetable broth. Whisk until the miso is completely dissolved.

2. Add in the cubed tofu, shiitake mushrooms, and scallions. Bring to a simmer and cook for 35 minutes.

3. Turn off the heat and stir in the sesame oil.

Serving Suggestions: Enjoy this soup as a light lunch or dinner with a side of toasted whole grain bread.

Egg Drop Soup

This soup includes both eggs and fresh veggies for a nutrientdense, fiberrich meal and excellent source of probiotic benefits for those with IBS.

Ingredients:

2 tablespoons olive oil

1/2 cup diced onion

2 cloves of garlic, minced

4 cups vegetable broth

2 tablespoons cornstarch

2 eggs, beaten

2 green onions, thinly sliced

Salt and pepper, to taste

Preparation Time: 15 minutes

Method of Preparation:

1. Begin by heating the olive oil in a medium pot on mediumhigh heat.

2. Add in the diced onion and minced garlic. Sauté for 23 minutes until fragrant.

3. Add the vegetable broth and bring to a simmer.

4. In a small bowl whisk together the cornstarch and eggs.

5. Slowly and steadily pour the egg mixture into the pot while stirring continuously.

6. Turn off the heat and stir in the green onions.

7. Taste and season with salt and pepper as needed.

Serving Suggestions: Enjoy this soup as a light lunch or dinner with a side of toasted whole grain bread.

Probiotic Veggie Wrap

This nutritious wrap includes a fiberfilled combination of probioticrich veggies and legumes for a beneficial meal option for those with IBS.

Ingredients:

2 whole wheat tortillas

2 slices swiss cheese

1/4 cup sauerkraut

1/2 cup cooked quinoa

1/4 cup roasted red peppers, diced

1/4 cup cucumber, diced

2 tablespoons hummus

Preparation Time: 10 minutes

Method of Preparation:

1. Begin by spreading hummus in the middle portion of the tortillas.

2. Layer the remaining ingredients on top of the hummus, starting with the swiss cheese, followed by the sauerkraut, cooked quinoa, roasted red peppers, and cucumber.

3. Roll the tortillas up and place the wrap in an oven toaster oven to melt the cheese, or in a skillet over medium heat to heat everything through.

4. Cut the wrap into smaller pieces before serving and enjoy!

Serving Suggestions: Enjoy this wrap as a light lunch or dinner with a side of roasted vegetables or a green salad.

Avocado Toast with Eggs

This meal is a great combination of protein and vitaminrich ingredients, such as avocado and eggs, making it an excellent option for those with IBS.

Ingredients:

1 small avocado, sliced

2 slices of whole wheat bread

2 eggs

Salt and pepper, to taste

Preparation Time: 10 minutes

Method of Preparation:

1. Begin by toasting the slices of whole wheat bread in a toaster oven or regular oven.

2. Once toasted, top each piece of bread with avocado slices.

3. In a small nonstick skillet, heat some olive oil over mediumhigh heat.

4. Crack the eggs into the skillet and season with salt and pepper. Cook the eggs until desired doneness.

5. Place the cooked eggs on top of the avocado slices and enjoy!

Serving Suggestions: Enjoy this toast as a light breakfast or lunch with a side of roasted vegetables or a green salad.

Sauteed Spinach and Mushrooms

Rich in vitamins and minerals, this meal is a nutrientpacked combination of fiberfilled mushrooms and spinach, making it a great choice for those with IBS.

Ingredients:

2 tablespoons olive oil

2 cloves of garlic, minced

1/2 cup sliced mushrooms

2 cups fresh spinach leaves

Salt and pepper, to taste

Preparation Time: 10 minutes

Method of Preparation:

1. Begin by heating the olive oil in a large skillet over mediumhigh heat.

2. Add the minced garlic and mushrooms. Sauté for 23 minutes until fragrant.

3. Add the spinach leaves and season with salt and pepper. Sauté for a few minutes until the spinach is wilted and cooked through.

Serving Suggestion: Enjoy this sauté as a side dish to your favorite meal.

Zucchini Frittata

Loaded with vitamins and minerals, this frittata is high in fiber and probioticrich, making it an ideal meal choice for those with irritable bowel syndrome.

Ingredients:

2 tablespoons olive oil

2 cloves of garlic, minced

1 small zucchini, cut into thin slices

3 eggs,beaten

1/4 cup Parmesan cheese

Salt and pepper, to taste

Preparation Time: 15 minutes

Method of Preparation:

1. Begin by heating the olive oil in a medium nonstick pan over mediumhigh heat.

2. Add the minced garlic and zucchini slices. Sauté for 23 minutes until lightly browned.

3. In a medium bowl, whisk together the eggs and Parmesan cheese.

4. Pour the egg mixture into the pan over the zucchini and season with salt and pepper.

5. Cook until the eggs are set, about 57 minutes.

Serving Suggestion: Enjoy this frittata as a light breakfast or lunch with a side of fresh fruit or a green salad.

Egg Omelet with Whole Wheat Bread

Enjoy this highprotein egg omelet accompanied by nutritious whole wheat bread for a meal that is beneficial for those with IBS.

Ingredients:

2 tablespoons olive oil

1 small onion, diced

2 cloves of garlic, minced

3 eggs, beaten

1/4 cup grated cheese

2 slices of whole wheat bread

Salt and pepper, to taste

Preparation Time: 10 minutes

Method of Preparation:

1. Begin by heating the olive oil in a medium nonstick pan over medium heat.

2. Add the diced onion and minced garlic. Sauté for 23 minutes until fragrant.

3. In a medium bowl, whisk together the eggs and Parmesan cheese.

4. Pour the egg mixture into the pan and season with salt and pepper.

5. Cook until the eggs are set, about 34 minutes.

6. Flip the omelet and cook for another 12 minutes.

7. Toast the slices of whole wheat bread in a toaster oven while the omelet cooks.

Serving Suggestion: Enjoy this omelet as a light breakfast or lunch with a side of fresh fruit or a green salad.

DINNER

Baked Salmon with Asparagus

Enjoy this healthy and flavorful baked salmon dish topped with asparagus. This dish is packed with Omega3 fatty acids, which helps reduce inflammation and is especially beneficial for IBS sufferers.

Ingredients:

4 salmon fillets

1 tsp of olive oil

1/2 tsp of lemon juice

2 cloves of garlic, minced

1/2 tsp of extra virgin olive oil

2 bunches of asparagus spears

Salt and pepper, to taste

Preparation Time: 25 minutes

Method of Preparation:

1. Preheat oven to 375 degrees Fahrenheit.

2. Place salmon fillets in a single layer in a lightly greased baking dish.

3. Drizzle with olive oil and lemon juice. Sprinkle with garlic

4. Place asparagus spears around the salmon. Drizzle with extra virgin olive oil and season with salt and pepper to taste.

5. Bake for 20-25 minutes or until salmon is cooked through.

Serving Suggestions: Serve with steamed or roasted potatoes, garlic bread, and/or a green salad.

Broiled Chicken with Steamed Veggies

Fill your plate with this combination of nutrientpacked steamed vegetables and juicy, flavorful broiled chicken. Low in fat and high in fiber, this dish is perfect for anyone suffering from IBS.

Ingredients:

2 tbsp of olive oil

1 tsp of minced garlic

1/2 tsp of rosemary

1/4 tsp of thyme

Salt and pepper, to taste

4 cups of assorted fresh vegetables (broccoli, carrots, green beans, etc)

Preparation Time: 30 minutes

Method of Preparation:

1. Preheat oven broiler to high.

2. Place chicken breasts in a baking dish. Drizzle with olive oil.

3. Sprinkle garlic, rosemary, thyme, salt and pepper on top of the chicken.

4. Place in oven on the middle rack and broil for 10 minutes. Flip the chicken over and broil an additional 10 minutes until cooked through.

5. Meanwhile, place vegetables in a steamer pot and steam for 8-10 minutes until cooked through.

Serving Suggestions: Serve with white or brown rice, a side of mashed potatoes, and/or roasted cauliflower.

Slow Cooker Turkey Chili

This hearty slow cooker turkey chili is packed full of flavor and nutrition. It contains antioxidants and antiinflammatory compounds which may help comfort IBS sufferers.

Ingredients:

1 lb of ground turkey

1 28 oz can of diced tomatoes

1 15 oz can of black beans

1 15 oz can of red kidney beans

1 cup of diced onion

2 cloves of garlic, minced

2 tbsp of chili powder

1 tsp of cumin

1 tsp of paprika

Salt and pepper, to taste

Preparation Time: 46 Minutes

Method of Preparation:

1. Place the turkey in a large slow cooker.

2. Add tomatoes, black beans, red kidney beans, diced onion, garlic, chili powder, cumin, paprika, salt and pepper to the slow cooker.

3. Stir all ingredients together and cover.

4. Cook on low heat until its done.

Serving Suggestions: Serve with warm tortilla chips, shredded cheese, plain Greek yogurt, and/or your favorite chili toppings.

Zucchini Noodles with Tomato Sauce

Enjoy this light and healthy meal of zucchini noodles and homemade tomato sauce. Low in fat and high in fiber, this dish is ideal for anyone with IBS.

Ingredients:

4 large zucchinis

1 tbsp of olive oil

2 cloves of garlic, minced

1 28 oz can of diced tomatoes

1 tsp of dried basil

1/2 tsp of dried oregano

Salt and pepper, to taste

Preparation Time: 25 minutes

Method of Preparation:

1. Using a spiralizer or julienne peeler, cut zucchinis into noodles.

2. Heat olive oil in a large skillet over medium heat. Add garlic and cook for a minute or two until fragrant.

3. Add diced tomatoes, basil, oregano, salt and pepper and simmer for 10-15 minutes.

4. Add zucchini noodles to the sauce and cook for 23 minutes until zucchini is just tender.

Serving Suggestions: Serve with warm garlic bread, Parmesan cheese, and/or horiatiki (Greek cucumber tomato salad).

Greek Egg & Vegetable Bake

This proteinpacked Greek egg & vegetable bake is loaded with nutrients and flavor. It contains gutfriendly probiotics and is great for soothing IBS symptoms.

Ingredients:

1 medium onion, chopped

1 bell pepper, deseeded and chopped

1 cup of fresh mushrooms, sliced

1/2 cup of marinated artichoke hearts, quartered

1 14 oz can of diced tomatoes

1/2 cup of fresh spinach, chopped

4 large eggs

1/2 cup of feta cheese

Salt and pepper, to taste

Preparation Time: 25 minutes

Method of Preparation:

1. Preheat oven to 350 degrees Fahrenheit. Grease a 9x13inch baking dish with olive oil.

2. Place onion, bell pepper, mushrooms, artichoke hearts, tomatoes, and spinach in the baking dish.

3. Crack eggs over the vegetables and mix them in. Sprinkle feta cheese over the top and season with salt and pepper to taste.

4. Bake in oven for 25 minutes until eggs are cooked through.

Serving Suggestions: Serve with warmed pita bread and/or tzatziki (yogurt cucumber dip).

Spinach & Cauliflower Risotto

Enjoy this creamy and comforting combination of spinach and cauliflower risotto. Loaded with gutfriendly ingredients, this dish helps to promote digestive health and is ideal for IBS sufferers.

Ingredients:

2 cups of vegetable broth

1 head of cauliflower, roughly chopped

2 cloves of garlic, minced

1 cup of frozen spinach

1/2 cup of freshly grated Parmesan cheese

1/4 cup of heavy cream

Salt and pepper, to taste

Preparation Time: 25 minutes

Method of Preparation:

1. Heat broth in a large pot over medium heat. Once hot, add cauliflower, garlic, and spinach. Cook for 57 minutes until cauliflower is just tender.

2. Reduce heat to low and add Parmesan cheese and cream. Stir until cheese is melted and combined.

3. Season with salt and pepper to taste.

Serving Suggestions: Serve with grilled chicken, a side of roasted vegetables, and/or a green salad.

Turkey & Vegetable Meatloaf

This flavorful turkey & vegetable meatloaf is low in saturated fat and high in fiber, which can help reduce IBS symptoms.

Ingredients:

1 lb of lean ground turkey

1/2 cup of diced onion

1/2 cup of diced bell pepper

1/2 cup of grated carrots

1/4 cup of fresh parsley, chopped

1/4 cup of bread crumbs (preferably glutenfree)

2 eggs, lightly beaten

2 cloves of garlic, minced

1 tsp of Worcestershire sauce

1/2 tsp of dried oregano

Salt and pepper, to taste

Preparation Time: 1 hour

Method of Preparation:

1. Preheat oven to 375 degrees Fahrenheit. Grease a large baking dish with nonstick cooking spray.

2. In a large bowl, combine turkey, onion, bell pepper, carrots, parsley, bread crumbs, eggs, garlic, Worcestershire sauce, oregano, salt and pepper. Use your hands to mix ingredients together until everything is evenly incorporated.

3. Transfer mixture to the prepared baking dish and shape into a loaf.

4. Bake for 45-60 minutes or until cooked through. Let cool for a few minutes before serving.

Serving Suggestions: Serve with mashed potatoes, a side of steamed broccoli, and/or garlic toast.

Broiled Cod with Herbed Brown Rice

Enjoy this savory and nutritious combination of broiled cod and herbed brown rice. This dish is packed with essential vitamins, minerals, and omega3 fatty acids to help reduce inflammation, an important benefit for IBS sufferers.

Ingredients:

4 cod fillets

1 tsp of olive oil

2 cloves of garlic, minced

1 tsp of dried oregano

Salt and pepper, to taste

3 cups of cooked brown rice

2 tbsp of fresh parsley, chopped

Preparation Time: 25 minutes

Method of Preparation:

1. Preheat oven broiler to high. Grease a baking dish with nonstick cooking spray.

2. Place cod fillets in the baking dish. Drizzle with olive oil and season with garlic, oregano, salt and pepper.

3. Broil in oven for 10 minutes or until fish is cooked through.

4. In a small saucepan, heat cooked brown rice with parsley and salt and pepper to taste.

Serving Suggestions: Serve with a side of ovenroasted vegetables, fresh lemon wedges, and/or a side salad.

Oven Roasted Turkey & Vegetables

This combination of ovenroasted turkey and vegetables is the perfect way to enjoy a flavorful and nutritious meal. Packed with vitamins, minerals, and antioxidants, this dish may help to ease IBS discomfort.

Ingredients:

1 lb of turkey breast, cut into bitesized cubes

1 red pepper, deseeded and chopped

1 zucchini, sliced

1/2 cup of cherry tomatoes

1/2 cup of mushrooms, sliced

1/4 cup of olive oil

2 cloves of garlic, minced

1 tsp of rosemary

Salt and pepper, to taste

Preparation Time: 25 minutes

Method of Preparation:

1. Preheat oven to 400 degrees Fahrenheit. Line a baking sheet with parchment paper.

2. Place turkey cubes, red pepper, zucchini, tomatoes, and mushrooms on the baking sheet.

3. Drizzle with olive oil and sprinkle with garlic, rosemary, salt and pepper.

4. Roast in oven for 20-25 minutes or until turkey is cooked through.

Serving Suggestions: Serve with roasted potatoes, rice pilaf, and/or a side of steamed green beans.

Roasted Vegetable & Tuna Salad

Enjoy this delicious salad of roasted vegetables and tuna. High in fiber and low in saturated fats, this salad is great for soothing IBS symptoms.

Ingredients:

1 red onion, sliced

2 large sweet potatoes, peeled and cut into cubes

1 red pepper, deseeded and chopped

2 cloves of garlic, minced

1 tbsp of olive oil

Salt and pepper, to taste

2 6oz cans of tuna, drained

1/2 cup of red wine vinegar

2 tbsp of honey

1/4 cup of fresh parsley, chopped

Preparation Time: 25 minutes

Method of Preparation:

1. Preheat oven to 400 degrees Fahrenheit. Line a baking sheet with parchment paper.

2. Place onion, sweet potatoes, red pepper, and garlic on the baking sheet. Drizzle with olive oil and season with salt and pepper to taste.

3. Roast in oven for 20-25 minutes until vegetables are tender.

4. Meanwhile, add tuna, red wine vinegar, honey, and parsley to a large bowl. Mix together until everything is combined.

5. Add roasted vegetables to the bowl and mix together. Serve immediately.

Serving Suggestions: Serve over a bed of arugula or spinach, with whole grain crackers, and/or a side of crusty bread.

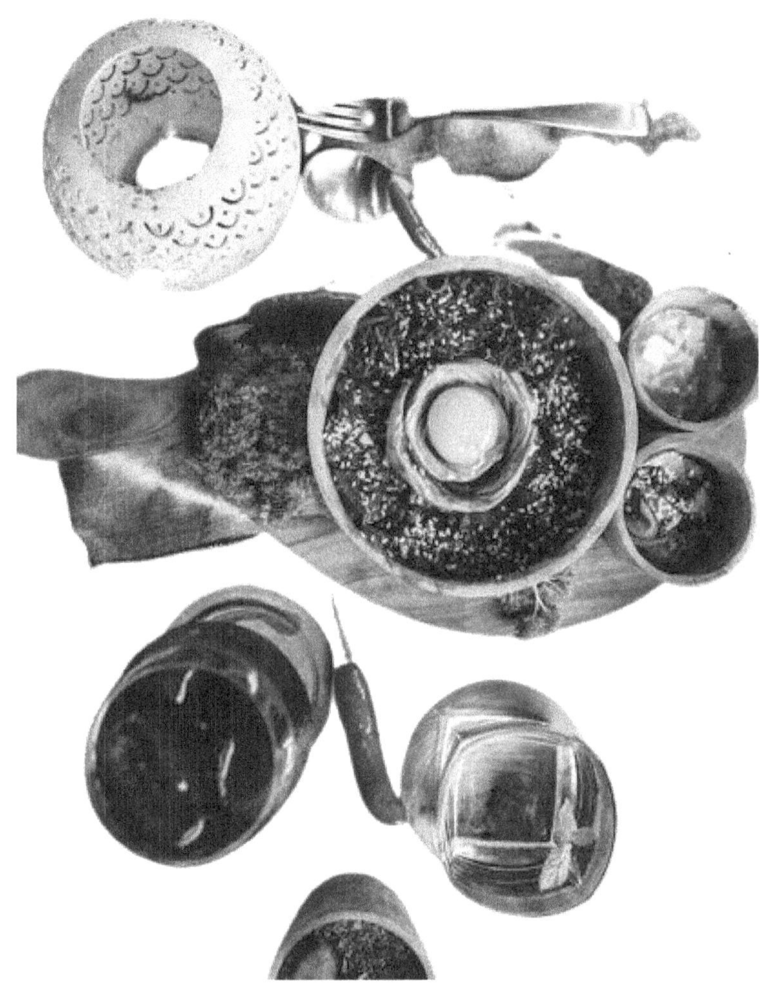

CONCLUSION

In conclusion, IBS Diet Cookbook for Beginners is more than just a collection of recipes; it's a guide to transforming lives and reclaiming control over one's digestive health.

Throughout these pages, you would have discovered that an IBS friendly diet does not mean sacrificing flavor or enjoyment.

Instead, it invites you to explore the rich tapestry of ingredients that can nourish your body and soothe your sensitive digestive systems.

I need you to embraced the notion that food can be both medicine and a source of comfort, bringing joy to your plates and relief to your bellies.

So go forth, embrace the possibilities that lie within your kitchen and continue to savor the flavors of life. With each meal you create, you are nourishing not only your body but also your spirit.

Trust in the transformative power of food and may your journey towards managing IBS be filled with joy, vitality, and a renewed sense of vitality.

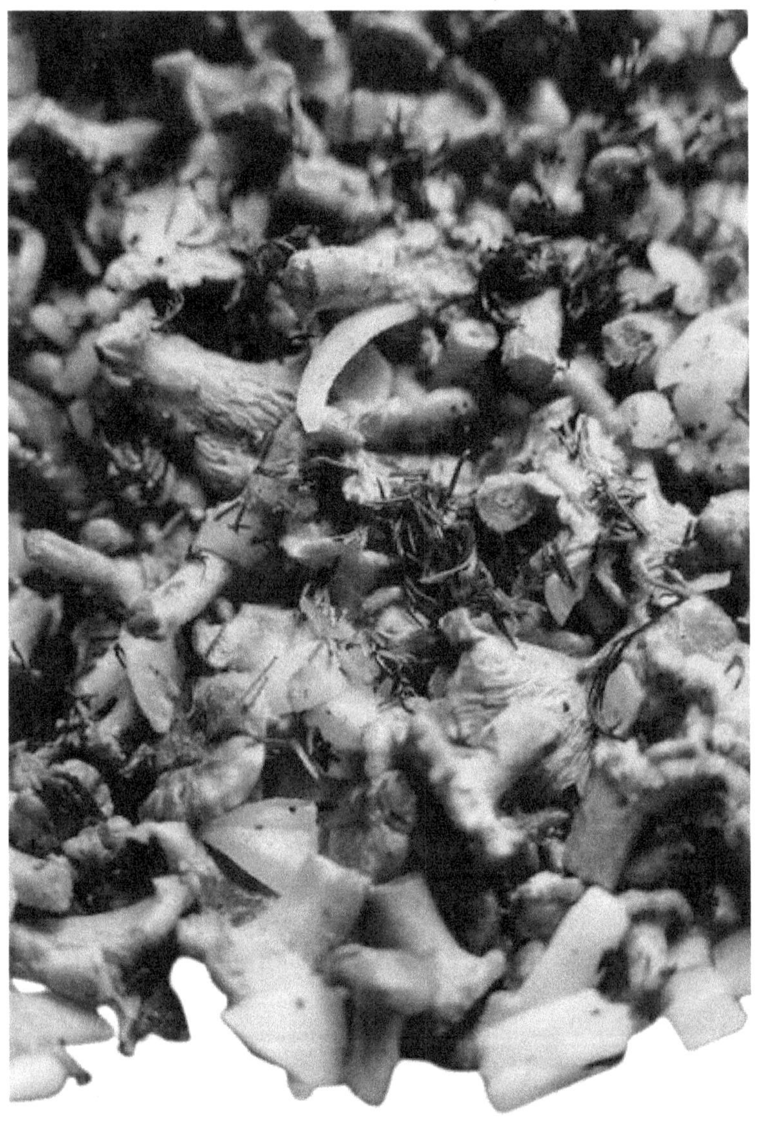